HOW TO CURE TENNIS ELBOW

How To Cure Tennis Elbow

The Definitive Guide For The Treatment of Tennis Elbow

Alan Nicholson

Copyright © 2013 by Alan Nicholson
ISBN-13: 978-1482334180
ISBN-10: 1482334186

All rights reserved. This book or any portion thereof may not be reproduced or used in any manner whatsoever without the express written permission of the publisher except for the use of brief quotations for the purpose of book reviews or articles, without the prior written permission of the publisher.

The information provided in this book is designed to provide helpful information on the subjects discussed. This book is not meant to be used, nor should it be used, to diagnose or treat any medical condition. For diagnosis or treatment of any medical problem, consult your own physician. The publisher and author are not responsible for any specific health or allergy needs that may require medical supervision and are not liable for any damages or negative consequences from any treatment, action, application or preparation, to any person reading or following the information in this book. References are provided for informational purposes only and do not constitute endorsement of any websites or other sources. Readers should be aware that the websites listed in this book may change.

TABLE OF CONTENT

CHAPTER 1 - THE PAIN OF TENNIS ELBOW 1

CHAPTER 2 - TENNIS ELBOW SYMPTOMS....5

CHAPTER 3 - TENNIS ELBOW DIAGNOSIS.. 17

CHAPTER 4 - TREATMENT TECHNIQUES TO MINIMIZE DAMAGE 21

- Pre-Game Techniques 24
- Techniques During Games 27
- After The Game Techniques 29

CHAPTER 5 - TENNIS ELBOW REHABILITATION 37

- Importance Of Rest 40
- Exercises To Do At Home 44
- Physical Therapy 50
- Using Your Insurance 54

CHAPTER 6 - PREVENTING A TENNIS ELBOW RELAPSE 55

    (A) TECHNIQUE MODIFICATIONS 57

    (B) EQUIPMENT MODIFICATIONS 60

    (C) COUNTERFORCE BRACES 64

CHAPTER 7 - PREVENT TENNIS ELBOW 67

FINAL NOTES ON TENNIS ELBOW 77

RESOURCE 1 - TENNIS ELBOW SECRETS 79

RESOURCE 2 - YOGA WELLNESS 80

Chapter 1 - The Pain Of Tennis Elbow

Rory was one of the top tennis players in his high school team. He was one of those players who oozes class and had a tennis scholarship awaiting him in college. Simon, meanwhile, was a forty-eight year old mechanic who works in the city when it happened to him. Madeline, a thirty year old racquetball player suffered the same consequences. It is the same for Jim, the sixty-five year old retiree and golf enthusiast.

All these people live in various parts of the world, come from different backgrounds but have one thing in common. They all suffer from the curse of tennis elbow. Do you think that tennis elbow only affects those people who play tennis? Nope, not at all.

Tennis elbow is a painful condition which affects anyone who uses their forearms, wrists or elbows repeatedly. Although it is known as 'tennis elbow', only around ten percent of the time that it affects the 'elbow'. Any person who uses their arms repeatedly throughout the day or during their hobby is prone to the curse of tennis elbow.

However, you need not worry. It doesn't mean that you must quit your job or stop doing the thing you love doing. With the right treatment plan on taking care of your condition, you can still go about your daily life normally.

The treatment of tennis elbow is something which contradicts many of the many medical practices in the United States. Many people assume that performing surgery would help them, but it doesn't.

Even rest isn't needed if you have this condition. You can be treated for tennis elbow while you are still active in your normal activities each day.

Tennis elbow is a condition which affects people of all walks of life. It is very painful and a doctor is required. The best doctors would be able to treat your tennis elbow condition with a non-surgical treatment plan.

Curing tennis elbow with the help of a good sports medicine doctor is very easy. They wouldn't prescribe any pills or perform any surgical procedures. The simple trick is to know the common symptoms and get the right diagnosis. From here, you are on the way to treating your painful condition.

Chapter 2 - Tennis Elbow Symptoms

With tennis elbow, the sufferer would feel several symptoms. All of them involves a certain pain around the elbow region. Among the pain a tennis elbow sufferer would feel includes:

(a) Pain When Holding Or Squeezing An Object

The pain around your elbow becomes worse when you hold or squeeze an object. This may include things like holding a racket or a golf club. If you find pain when holding it, there is a high possibility that you have tennis elbow.

Check if this is a one-time occurrence or something that happens continuously. If this happens continuously, look for a diagnosis. The pain may even get worse when you try to turn a doorknob or open a jar.

(b) Soreness Or Pain When Bending The Wrist

Many people confuse tennis elbow with the carpal tunnel syndrome. Both of them are completely different. When you have tennis syndrome, there would be certain soreness or pain which radiates from the forearm when you bend your wrist. The pain from tennis elbow is more than an ache than a shooting pain. It would get worse over time if you ignore it.

(c) Pain Or Tenderness Around Your Elbow's Bony Part

This is perhaps the most common symptom of tennis elbow. However, just because you have this symptom doesn't necessarily mean that you have tennis elbow. The symptoms of tennis elbow are similar to other forms of symptoms or condition.

This type of pain could also be because of a contusion. If the pain persists however, there is a high possibility that you suffer from tennis elbow. There is a way to determine if you have a contusion.

When you hit your elbow and there's a black and blue spot in the area, high possibility is that you have contusion. The pain also wouldn't subside and you should see a doctor immediately.

(d) Pain In Arm When Your Wrist Is Extended

This is another common symptom that you would have when you have tennis elbow. The pain would be excruciating and you would find it hard to even write sometimes.

Anyone who has this symptom may find that their arms won't hurt if they slightly bend it. Therefore, they try to keep their arms from being extended. However, this is only a temporary relief.

(e) Weak Grip In Your Hands

Those who have tennis elbow may only notice it when they realize they have such a weak grip. They may realize it when they shake their hands or turn open a door knob. This would prompt a trip to the doctor immediately.

Again, those symptoms can mirror other conditions and this make diagnosis so important.

****

While these symptoms are extremely painful, most people don't normally seek treatment straight away. Among those people that come for tennis elbow research, all of them seek treatment but not all came for the right treatment. With the right treatment plan, you may need up to six weeks and your elbow would be like brand new. During the meantime, you could still perform your activities.

If you seek assistance from the doctor too late, there is a possibility that your condition might be worse. Many come to a doctor only after they have tried other forms of treatment. They have gotten the wrong diagnosis before and others have treated it seriously only when they are told they need surgery.

Most people wouldn't rush to a doctor straight away after experiencing pain in their elbow. When you perform any repetitive movements with your arms or elbow, be aware of the possible symptoms of tennis elbow and know what to look for. Tennis elbow shouldn't scare you as more than 90% of cases can be cured with six weeks of physical therapy.

On the other side, there are other symptoms that may not be caused by tennis elbow. They may be caused by a more serious condition that would need instant medical intervention. The symptoms include:

- **Continuous Pain For More Than A Week.** This could be because of tennis elbow as well but it could be because of other form of pain. If the pain persists, you should talk to your doctor immediately about it. This is imperative if your pain gets worse.

- **Excruciating Pain That Wakes You Up In Your Sleep.** The pain from tennis elbow may be very painful but they won't wake you up. A pain that wakes you up from sleep should be examined me a doctor immediately.
- **Unable To Bend Your Wrist.** When you have trouble bending your wrist without feeling any pain, it is an indication that there is a more serious condition. You could even have a broken wrist or a fracture. Talk to your doctor immediately.
- **Bruising.** Bruises around your arms or wrist are a strong indication that you are having a contusion or fracture. You should seek your doctor's advice about it. Bruising or swelling could indicate that a contusion or fracture. Simply put, a contusion is what happens when you bang your arm against something

hard. From the bang, you would get a blue and black mark. If the swelling doesn't go, check with your doctor immediately.

- **Losing Your Grip.** When you lose your grip on doorknobs or you start to drop things, it is an indication that you suffer from a more serious illness. You shouldn't ignore it. If this happen repeatedly, you may suffer from other condition like carpal tunnel syndrome.

To cure tennis elbow, you need to recognize the symptoms and not ignore them. Very often, those people who have symptoms and hope they will go away. We don't want to go to the doctor for each pain that we have. However, you should seek a doctor if there a persistent problems.

I have seen patients who wait till until a year until the seek treatment. Some of those patients use aspirin to relieve the pain and don't really enjoy their activities.

The point in this is such. While you don't have to seek a doctor every time you experience some pain, if you feel pain from doing certain repetitive movement on a consistent basis, you should realize that you have a risk of developing tennis elbow.

It isn't a serious condition and you shouldn't be worried about it. If you take steps to cure this syndrome becomes the pain becomes too excruciating, you will cure it and enjoy a better quality of life.

Be clear that only a doctor can diagnose if you have tennis elbow. You may have the symptoms mentioned in the earlier parts of this book, but if you feel that you have tennis elbow, seek a doctor immediately and get the right diagnosis once and for all.

When seeking a doctor to cure your suspected tennis elbow, you should find someone who specializes in sports. Don't just seek the normal general practitioner as they wouldn't be the right people.

What To Tell Your Doctor

When you experience the symptoms, be careful to note when it started and if they get worse over time. You should also be clear about the symptoms that you have, if the pain becomes worse and other common symptoms.

Take note of other symptoms as well. This may include numbness in your hands, headaches, forgetfulness or any loss of sensation. The specialized doctor would ask you certain questions, so it would be better to write down any symptoms that you feel during the period to ensure that your doctor can diagnose you better.

Be clear that tennis elbow need not be crippling. It isn't life threatening at all but could heavily interfere with your life. Learn more about how to cure this condition in the next few chapters.

Chapter 3 - Tennis Elbow Diagnosis

To be clear again, only a doctor can rightly tennis elbow. Don't waste your time reading the internet or books to diagnose it yourself. This book merely serves to assist with understanding the pain that you have and giving you possible treatment methods.

Self-diagnosis is a total waste of time. The doctor can easily diagnose this condition just from performing a simple physical examination on your arm and elbow.

The doctor would ask several questions to ensure that is the right diagnosis. He would examine your arm, stretch it and ask you where hurts. There is very little possibilities that an x-ray or blood work is needed. However, he may decide to play it safe if they feel you are suffering from a condition which is even worse than tennis elbow. The doctor would want to know the following:

- If you have any pain or conditions that should be of concern?
- What activity or job you have that you do on a regular basis?
- When you first notice the condition?
- Does the pain radiate - Tell the doctor when your pain starts and ends?
- Does the pain keep you awake at night?

Some doctors would test your grip and another careful examination and if everything is confirmed, only then would he diagnose you with tennis elbow. It is extremely important that this is done rightly as you wouldn't want to be diagnosed wrongly.

This is why it is important to find a sports medicine doctor. They have seen plenty of tennis elbow cases and would be able to make a quicker diagnosis.

Once it is confirmed, seek for a treatment plan with your doctor immediately. If there is a specialized treatment plan, you should start it right away. The doctor may choose to send you to a physical therapist or another doctor who specialize with this condition.

Without a doubt, a doctor who specializes in sports medicine for tennis elbow treatment is better. This is because this isn't a condition which only affects a small group of people. It is very common in the United States, affecting more than ten million people each year. Although this condition isn't caused by sports alone, it is still considered a sports injury. It is best treated by those in sports medicine.

Make sure you get the right and thorough diagnosis from a qualified doctor before starting your treatment with the physical therapist or doctor. Don't worry too much about the cost as getting a diagnosis is as simple as a doctor visit. Should you suspect you have tennis elbow, always look for a sport medicine doctor as quickly as you can.

Chapter 4 - Treatment Techniques To Minimize Damage

Once you are diagnosed with tennis elbow, you don't need to stop your daily activities that you love. Rehabilitation is something to consider for the future. However, you can still play tennis, golf or work normally, if you use the right techniques.

When you use these techniques to alleviate the pain, you may be able to arrest it. The moment you are pain-free, you could undergo a more detailed rehabilitation process which cures your condition for good, once and for all.

However, most doctors would still recommend a rest in order to cure tennis elbow once and for all. Tennis elbow is caused by elbow tendon tears. A tear in tendon happens because of an overuse or improper use of your tendons.

Rest could heal your overused tendons and cure the problem for the long term, but it may not be the most practical way. Some people depend on their arms to work or play a sport. Therefore, it could be very difficult to take time off from work for a long period.

There are people who play tennis for a living or those people who work as carpenters. These people use a great deal of their hands. People who are self-employed would be forced to continue working to ensure they could provide money for their family. It isn't sufficient to live on social security disability and if you really succumb to tennis elbow, you may not be able to work for a full year.

A professional tennis player may have a full season of tennis waiting for him and he just can't afford to stop playing midway through the season. Professional athletes are prone to this condition and it wouldn't be feasible to stop their game. For example, they may have scheduled to play in a certain tournament and have to continue playing because it's their likelihood. They need to endure great pain while playing the game.

In the following chapters, there are techniques which you can use before, during and after your tennis game that would help you. They would assist you in alleviating the pain and allow play to continue, although you suffered from the tennis elbow symptoms.

Pre-Game Techniques

Before playing any sports, one should take anti-inflammatory drug like ibuprofen or naproxen. Nonsteroidal anti-inflammatory drugs, usually abbreviated to NSAIDs, would help you alleviate some pain. This enables you to perform better.

Using this drug on a long term basis would have side effects however. According to research, using NSAIDs is linked to digestive problems. Don't ever rely on NSAIDs for too long a period as they would cause ulcers or stomach problems. Even taking a couple of Tylenol before a tennis match would be very helpful just doesn't take them on a long term basis.

Besides medication, one should also do some arm stretching before your match. You should stretch your shoulders, forearms, biceps and triceps before the start of play. Of course, you should stretch regardless of whether you have a tennis elbow condition or not.

Many people experience sports injuries because they don't spend time warming up or stretching properly before playing their game. Make it a point to stretch always before your play any sports whatsoever.

Don't neglect your legs. You may not feel any pain in your legs at present, but you wouldn't want anything else to happen to them.

Make sure that you have proper circulation in your arms. Warm up using hand stretching techniques. This is done with a serious of arm warmers. Warm ups are important in improving your circulation while you are playing and this would ensure that you wouldn't suffer too much from the effects of your tennis elbow.

Make it a point to also wear arm warmers during your warm up as it helps to keep your hands warm.

Techniques During Games

While playing the game, you should use a counterforce elastic band that helps relieve the pain in your elbow. It has helped many people who suffer from this condition. You could get such a band from sporting shops or through online stores.

Another thing to consider for tennis players is to ensure that they aren't holding their racquets to tightly. Take a look at how you hold your racquet. Check how heavy your racquet is. You should also try to learn the right grip to hold. Loosen up or use one which is of the lighter weight, it would help with your tennis elbow condition. This allows the pain to subside.

If you feel like you are holding the racquet right, then find for a lighter racquet which you are more comfortable with. Search for sports shops or seek online recommendations on racquets which are not too heavy for you. It may cost more, but it's worth it.

Warming bands around your elbows would also help you tremendously. Wrists bands are also a great help if you feel comfortable wearing them. When your tendons are warm while you play your sport, the lower probability of you aggravating your tennis elbow condition.

You can find elbow bands or wrist bands in just about any sports shop. If you are an avid tennis player, it's most certain that you have seen people wearing them. This goes a long way in ensuring that their tendons and muscles are warm and in great operating condition.

After The Game Techniques

After the game, it is normal that you want to rush home and celebrate. However, you would need to recover from your exercise so that you are in good condition to play well in your next match. For this, I would recommend a healing method called "PRICE". It is an acronym for Protection, Rest, Ice, Compression and Elevation.

(a) Protect Your Arm

After your sporting activity, it's the best time to protect your arm from any activity that further aggravates your painful tennis elbow condition. There is no need for any bandage or to put it in a sling. However, you would want to rest instead of doing something else that would further aggravate your condition. You already need to use your hands for your main event (like work or sports). As such you wouldn't want to 'waste' energy on things which would further aggravate your problem.

Don't further use your hands if you don't need to. Save it up for your 'main' event. Protecting your arm from further injury so you could continue to enjoy other activities you enjoy or what you do for a living.

(b) Rest Your Arm

Take some resting time after your activities. In fact, give your entire body some rest after a big match. Remember that you have spent a lot of your energy on your bid workout and it is now time to rest and allow it to heal. After a tennis game, you should rest your arm properly.

Rest doesn't mean that you just take naps, but it means that you should restrict your movement to give your body the rest it deserves. Avoid any strenuous activities as it allows your tendon to repair and alleviate the pain.

(c) Ice Your Arm

This is often a very contentious issue. Many doctors believe it wouldn't help at all. Some doctors believe that you should use heat when you have pain while some recommend using ice.

What ice does is that it would help reduce the swelling and alleviate the pain from the tennis elbow. Get your icepack and hold it up to your arms for about an hour after your game. This greatly reduces the pain in your arm and your arm would feel much better.

(d) Compression

If the pain is very severe, you can look to use compression. This may include bandaging your arms. Use an ACE bandage and ensure that it is immobile. This isn't necessary but work extremely well if you have severe pain. Keep your arm compressed for about two days after playing a tennis match or after a game of golf.

(e) Elevation

In severe tennis elbow cases, elevation is often recommended. This involves keeping your arm immobile and elevated on a pillow or other comfortable object. However, this isn't recommended if your tennis elbow isn't severe. In many cases, your pain can be easily alleviated when you protect your arm, rest it and by using an ice pack. From here, you would feel great and be ready to play immediately.

****

When you experience any pain, many doctors provide pain medication. Although tennis elbow is an extremely painful condition, don't depend solely on over the counter medication. Medications only play the role of a painkiller. Don't be overly dependent on medication.

There are two main kinds of pain medication. They include over-the-counter medications and prescription pain medications.

(1) Over-The-Counter Pain Medications

NSAIDs are great to use on a shorter term basis. Take a couple of ibuprofen when you have a headache, backache or other pain from playing a sport and you would feel better instantly. However, if you use it on a long term basis, it would be extremely helpful for your digestive system and could even cause stomach cancer. It would also cause stomach ulcers and liver damage. If you are in a habit of constantly using this sort of medication, seek a doctor and find another alternative therapy for your pain.

(2) Prescription Pain Medications

The most common form of prescription pain medication is Vicodin. The moment you mention the word 'pain' to your doctor and they would immediately prescribe Vicodin.

Many doctors have stopped prescribing Oxycontin because it has known to be a drug that you could be addicted to. Therefore, Vicodin is more widely prescribed when dealing with pain. Other drugs like Tylenol and Codeine are addictive and have long term serious side effects. There would be difficult withdrawal symptoms the moment you stop taking it.

Always remember that pain relievers or medications are merely to mask the pain. They won't eliminate the real cause of the pain. It merely masks them to ensure that you won't feel the pain. You shouldn't use it on a long term pain for any pain whatsoever.

Pain medications are very addictive, to a point that people fake their pain in order to get doctor's prescriptions. Always remember that all these medications have very serious side effects and you shouldn't rely on them to deal with your pain from tennis elbow.

Look instead for a way to cure your condition. I am talking about rehabilitation. This would be discussed in the next chapter. This rehabilitation process has worked for many people. However, whatever that is discussed can alleviate pain. This PRICE technique would conquer your tennis elbow condition and control it better.

Chapter 5 - Tennis Elbow Rehabilitation

Ninety percent of tennis elbow sufferers would not need any form of surgery to cure it. It is completely rational to cure tennis elbow using normal treatment prescribed in the previous chapter. Using rest, flexibility and strengthening exercises; many people could easily cure tennis elbow.

The moment you are diagnosed with this condition, you need to ensure that your rehabilitation process starts straight away to ensure a faster cure. You may not be able to start the process immediately, but try to start it as soon as you can. After rehabilitation, your elbow would be as good as new. With a six week to three months procedure, you would be able to cure your tennis elbow once and for all.

Before starting your rehab process, you need to be pain-free. This is achieved by resting your arm as described from the previous chapter. This would ensure your arms are fully rested and free from pain. It may be tough for you, but stopping your daily activities helps speed up the process of pain alleviation. This rest period gives your tendon the time to heal.

As tennis elbow is a condition resulting from a torn tendon, you should ensure that your tendon is fully heal to ensure that the rehab process goes on smoothly. You should also ensure that your hand has a full range of motion and it returns to normal activity. Most of the time, this may not be completely possible. You still depend on your hands on your daily activities but try to start your rehab quickly to ensure you get a faster cure.

The success and speed of your healing depends a lot on your general health and your age. Those who are younger are able to heal faster. However, most people would be completely cured from their tennis elbow condition within two months. To put it in short, if you want to recover well with rehab, you need to rest well first.

Importance Of Rest

When you are "resting" for your tennis elbow, it doesn't mean that you can't do anything with your arm. However, it does mean that you avoid any repeated motion that would aggravate your condition. Before starting on any form of exercises prescribed in the previous chapter, make sure that your arm is free from pain. This helps your tennis elbow cure easier.

When it comes to alleviating the pain, cold generally works better than heat. Put a cold compressor on your arm once each day. After that, wait a few weeks before you start on the rehab process. Your severity affects how long you should be resting. If your condition is worst, the rest should be longer. As such, it is important to consult a physical therapist to assist you with this condition and advise you with the rehab process. They would give you the right instruction and what to do for preparing for rehab.

The rehab process could also be helped by a sport medicine doctor. They would generally be the one who is experienced with your condition. Remember that rehabilitation isn't just about getting back to your normal condition.

You also needs to learn how to fix things that aggravate your condition. This may include how your wrongly hold your racquet or golf clubs. You should also make stretching a habit.

Don't ever underestimate the power of resting your tendon. This helps ensure that your tendon is complete heal before using any form of rehab exercises for strengthening your tendon. Only when your tendon is completely healed and there is no pain do you begin the second part of the rehabilitation process. Don't get into the error of thinking that the moment you are free from any pain, you wouldn't need rehab.

This is something that actually aggravates most conditions. When you still have this condition, all this would just cure it for a while. You feel pain-free but the pain would still arise next time when you play the game. The suffering would come up again and again, until you are completely cured from this tennis elbow condition. This makes the tendon longer and longer to heal.

You should be clear that most people would ultimately need to have surgery to fix their tennis elbow condition. Many people have had a long history of tennis elbow and don't do anything about it. They may just take a rest, pain relievers or icing their arms. However, this normally isn't sufficient.

Even worse, some people don't even get a proper diagnosis for their condition. Don't ever let this happen to you. If you feel like you have any symptoms of it, seek proper diagnosis and treatment immediately.

Exercises To Do At Home

As you start out with your tennis elbow rehab, your physical therapist would need you to go to the clinic on a periodic basis. This ranges from once to twice a week. However, the therapist would also give you certain exercises that you could do from the comfort of your home.

This allows you to get a full range of motion with your hands. Practice these exercises as taught by your doctor so you could regain full use of your hand motions without suffering too much from the pain.

Before you start out, make sure that you are resting well and your doctor gives you the right steps to start out with your exercises. You would want to start out slowly and then slowly build up the exercises. This helps regain strength in your arms. Generally speaking, practice these exercises on both arm even if only one elbow is suffering from this condition. It doesn't hurt if you strengthen both arms.

One of the best ways to strengthen your hands (and biceps) is by lifting weights. However, you shouldn't life weights which are too heavy. Start out by lifting light weights like two pounds ones first. Using weights allows you to achieve a full range of motion with your hands.

When you are lifting weights, there shouldn't be any pain. The main purpose isn't to grow muscles but to strengthen the tendons in your arms. That is the reason why light weights are only used and that why you should start out slowly.

However, don't start using weights unless you can move your arm freely without experiencing any pain. Carrying weight should be as effortless as possible. When starting out, do about ten repetition of about five set per day. That might be nothing for you, but the key is to start out small. This is more than enough. Look to increase the repetition or sets after a week of doing it.

If you feel any pain during your weight exercises, you should stop doing it straight away. Weight exercises are to help you get back to using your arms in full range without feeling pain.

This would also strengthen your hand muscles. Ask your doctor's advice about how to use those weights and the proper exercise for you.

Range Of Motion Exercises

Besides using weights to build up the strength in your tendons, you can also use range of motion exercises to strengthen your tendons even more. Many sufferers have a problem when they extend their arms fully. This is because of the pain in their elbow tendon. Therefore, these exercises help extend your arm.

These exercises are incredibly simple to perform. One main exercise is one which you extend your arms as far out as possible slowly. From here, bend your elbow slowly. Do this for a minimum of eight repetition each day. Your arm would feel less stiff after a while.

Another form of exercise you could do if to gently life your arms over your head and then bring it to your side. Do this from the side and from the front of your body. It may feel stiff, but you would slowly loosen up and it becomes easy. Besides that, you can also perform a circular motion with your arms. Simply move your arms forward and then slowly move it backwards.

Racquet Exercises

Once you are done with the range of motion exercises, you could also practice with your racquet or golf club swings. Firstly, you need to learn how to properly hold your racquet or golf club. Learn from a professional. From here, you should lightly swing them in a motion that allows you to use it again. Ask your doctor for advice about how to do it right and how it causes less impact on your elbow tendons.

Gripping Exercises

Most people who suffer from tennis elbow have pain in their arms. This pain is so intense until holding a doorknob becomes very difficult. To strengthen your muscles in your arm, you can simply do it by gripping a squeeze ball and then gently releasing it. You can use a squash ball if you want.

This exercise is great for both your hands and strengthens your hands and wrists muscles. Ask your doctor for recommendation on the right exercise ball to use. With the right methods, you would learn how to grip better with your fingers. The purpose of these exercises is to strengthen your tendons in the elbow to ensure that your tennis elbow condition doesn't relapse.

Such practices should be always done with your doctor's instruction. These exercises are a few that your therapists would ask you to perform. Together with physical therapy, they would ensure that your hands become stronger and ready for other activities.

Physical Therapy

There are many rehabilitation centers around the United States which specialized in sport medicine. Among the services they offer is physical therapy. To cure tennis elbow, physical therapy can be performed from the comfort of your sports doctor's office or your physical therapist's office.

Most physical therapy is more than just the exercises in your therapist's office. There would be some instructions for you to perform at home. The amount of physical therapy and the length of it depend a lot on the damage that has been done on your tendon. Therapy is the sole treatment to treat tennis elbow and it is incredibly effective. No surgery is required.

Your physical therapist uses different techniques which is used to nimble your tendon and allows you to stretch it.

There would be a series of stretching exercises ad therapy that would help massage your tendon and the arm muscles. Besides stretching and therapy, you can also look to perform ice therapy or heating treatments. However, the focus would be on stretching your tendons without breaking. That is the main purpose of physical therapy.

Your physical therapist would teach you the right methods to exercise before you start any home-based exercise. This is to ensure that you wouldn't overstretch your tendons and how to perform the exercises correctly.

This is to ensure that you wouldn't further injure yourself. They may want you to practice these exercises in the therapist's office before they send you home.

You would need to be disciplined in this physical therapy part of rehabilitation. It is very tempting for you to feel that you have fully recovered as their elbow isn't bothering them.

The tendency is for them to quit the therapy halfway. Most of the time, the pain would still affect them after a certain period. Therefore, you should always finish physical therapy until the therapist say you are completely healed. Only then can you fully enjoy your activities.

Remember that physical therapy is more than ensuring that your arms could be used fully, it helps you prevent a future relapse of your tennis elbow condition. Anyone who has tennis elbow would eventually have a relapse, until they have made the appropriate changes as to how they approach their activities. You need to train yourself to be more flexible and rehab plays an important role in that.

As you religiously follow the physical therapy and follow what the doctor say, it is guaranteed that you can cure your tennis elbow condition without any surgery or medication.

This works in more than 90% of cases. Even if you have long faced such pain from tennis elbow, you don't need surgery at all. Follow this treatment plan accordingly by using flexibility and strengthening exercises and you would recover in a few weeks' time.

Using Your Insurance

The cost of curing tennis elbow may be prohibitive for certain people. However, if your injury is caused by your work, you could get a workmen's compensation. This would help pay for your treatment and pay for your time off work. To do this, there would be a need to file a workmen's compensation claim.

If you are an athlete and the injury is caused by certain sports, your insurance would still cover outpatient physical therapy. However, this needs to be prescribed by your doctor. As such, you should seek a proper doctor and ask him for a letter of recommendation. This is not a serious condition, but the rehabilitation process may be costly if you don't have proper insurance coverage. Therefore, seek insurance advice before starting out anything.

Chapter 6 - Preventing A Tennis Elbow Relapse

After going through your rehabilitation process and your doctor has gave you the permission to continue with your normal activities, there are certain things to keep in mind.

This is important to prevent a relapse of your condition. To ensure this, you would need certain modifications in order to prevent a relapse. This includes a technique or equipment modification.

In many situations, the cause of tennis elbow is because they have used equipment wrongly or simply used the wrong equipment.

If you continue doing the same thing after you have fully recovered, it is a high possibility that you would face the same problems after that. In this chapter, you would learn how to reduce the chances of you having tennis elbow.

56

(a) Technique Modifications

From professional golfers to tennis players, all of them change their techniques to ensure that they play better. Most of the time, this is because of a certain strain that they are feeling on their tendons and muscles. Legendary tennis player Roger Federer has changed the way he approached certain shots throughout the years. This modification in techniques helps his body cope better with the strain on his body.

When you swing your club/racquet, do you feel the pain?

Do you feel any discomfort from your swing?

Professional athletes constantly look for methods to improve their technique in a way that would put less stress on their body. Imagine professional athletes who have to hit thousands of shots a day. It puts an incredible stress on their body and having the right technique means you would be able to do it easier. This is not just for professional athletes but for recreational ones as well.

This is the importance of having proper technique. The beauty about having proper techniques is that you can do something easily and effortlessly. It's not just about doing it effectively; it's also about doing it efficiently. That's what technique is all about.

Trust me, it would be very tough for anyone to change to a new technique. This is similar to all forms of sports. Change is very difficult for anyone, especially if you have played a sport for a long period. But after a certain period, once you get the hook of the new technique, you would especially love it.

This technique change is a habitual change. It is difficult but it helps prevent the pain from tennis elbow from coming back. You should look at professional athletes like Roger Federer or Tiger Woods; who make millions of dollars from their swing. They realize the importance of having proper technique and so do you.

(b) Equipment Modifications

Another way of preventing the relapse of tennis elbow is to modify the equipment that you use. For tennis players, this may be using a lighter racquet or a lighter golf club for golfers. There are also other form of modifications which would help make it easier for you to swing better.

Try not to use too heavy equipment if you have tennis elbow. Many tennis players like using heavier racquets because if gives their shots extra power. However, if you have tennis elbow, this is a sacrifice that you must make. With a lighter tennis racquet, you may need to sacrifice power, but it prevents a relapse of your tennis elbow condition.

Besides the weight of your racquet, you should also use the right string tension. Talk to your professional sports shop owner and ask him to give you some advice. Understand the different strings that are available. Are you using a natural gut, nylon or polyurethane? Make sure not to use polyurethane strings.

It is highly recommended to use natural gut as it is the best string substance. It is the softest and allow the greatest flexibility. If you can't find natural gut, the second best would be using nylon or synthetic gut. Prevent using hard strings as it would cause an excessive impact on your racquet. You may end up hurting your hand and aggravating your tennis elbow.

Besides the type of string, the other important thing to consider is the tension of your strings. Some people string too tightly. It may give them more power, but it creates more vibrations on your racquet - something you wouldn't want.

After that, the factor you should consider is the size of the racquet head. Don't use a racquet which has too big a head as it would create more strain on your elbows. Find a racquet with a standard head size. The grip is also another main factor. If you choose a grip which is too big or small, it would also affect your wrist when you hit with it. This puts additional strain on your elbows.

One great thing to do is to bring your racquet to your sports medicine doctor to evaluate. See what alterations can be done to fit you better. Even golfers may alter their equipment to prevent a relapse of their tennis elbow. Many golfers do their elbows harm because they use clubs which are too heavy or of the wrong measurement. When you switch to a lighter club, you get a more comfortable grip and prevent a relapse of your condition.

In deciding if a club or racquet suits you, you can just feel it on your hand and arms as you swing them. If you feel it is too heavy and uncomfortable, you are most probably using the wrong equipment. An instant change is recommended. Remember that your equipment plays the main role. Your swing should be effortless and easy.

If you feel overstrained from using it, it is the wrong equipment. Once you have fully recovered from your tennis elbow, take a closer look at your sports equipment and make any necessary changes. It may take some time or cause a bit of money, but it is necessary so that you will enjoy the game for a long period of time.

(c) Counterforce Braces

Another great way that helps prevent a tennis elbow relapse is by using counterforce braces. These are used to lessen the strain on your elbows. Counterforce braces are strapped on your arm, below the elbow. This is to ensure that the tension is absorbed instead of affecting the elbow. This brace compresses the muscles and prevent it from expanding.

Counterforce braces wouldn't restrict your arm movements while you are playing any sports. This is very common among professional golfers. If technique modification and equipment modifications have been tried, then using braces is an alternative that you should try.

These braces can be found in many places, including sports shops and online stores.

****

Whether you are considering a modification in your technique, equipment or wearing a brace, you need to change your habits after you have finished the recovery process. This would prevent a future relapse. If you have suffered from tennis elbow last time, you would suffer again until you change your habits.

There is a way to prevent tennis elbow. This would be discussed in the next chapter.

Chapter 7 - Prevent Tennis Elbow

Although tennis elbow is often considered a sports injury, many people who use heavy equipment or hands repetitively are also prone to this condition. Tennis elbow surgery is something uncommon and only happens in less than ten percent of cases.

Surgery is only necessary when other forms of treatment methods have failed to work. However, through my experience, the tennis elbow treatment that I share in the beginning of this book is more than sufficient to ensure treatment. I have rarely seen a situation so severe that surgery is needed. Severe cases only happen on those who have neglected their condition for too many years.

Should you be required to for surgery to repair your elbow tendon, there is a high possibility that it wouldn't be the same. Injuries are such, the moment you have injured yourself, it wouldn't be the same. After surgery, you need to rest and rehabilitation period. This is the same thing even if you didn't have surgery in the first place.

However, I recommend that you try an intensive physical therapy period before trying surgery. Surgery changes your elbow and most sports doctors wouldn't even recommend it in the first place. Therefore, preventing it from happening again is very important. There are several things that would help prevent tennis elbow, which includes:

(a) Stretch Before Games

Before starting your sport, it is very important to stretch your arm and leg muscles. Those who have taken aerobics would know how to stretch and limber up before starting your exercise activity. Professional athletes know the same thing also.

Not stretching before games is only a mistake done by amateur or recreational athletes. This causes a tension in your arms and legs. As such, your muscles are strained and your tendons can be torn. This is why stretching is so important. Before playing any sports whatsoever, always warm up first.

(b) Exercise Your Arms

You can make your arms stronger by exercising them. Use the same exercises that you do when you are in the rehabilitation for tennis elbow.

Many people don't care too much about their body and think that their body would be strong forever. However, this is rarely the case.

Once you get older, you realize that your body start to weaken. Tennis elbow is a condition that could strike anyone, regardless of your age. You should use exercises well to ensure that you prevent tennis elbow. It would not only strengthen your arms but also your tendons.

(c) Equipment Modification

Take time to ensure that you are using the appropriate equipment. It is very important that you use the right golf club, tennis racquet or work equipment. This is to ensure that the minimum strain is placed on your elbow.

Make sure that your golf clubs and tennis elbow is easy for you to swing. In the previous chapter, I have already shared the kind of strings and tension that you should use to ensure that it wouldn't put unnecessary strain on you.

(d) Take Lessons

It helps a lot to take a lesson on the sport you are playing. Too many people play tennis or golf without going for lessons which teach them how to swing properly. Without taking lessons, you can end up damaging your body. This is especially common among golfers.

Many people play a certain sports but because of their lack of training, they develop bad swinging habits. This would not only harm your game, but your body as well.

Therefore, you should look to invest in some lessons if you really love the game. A lesson would teach you the right way to hold a golf club or racquet. Having the right technique not only allows you to enjoy the game more, but help prevent your condition from relapsing.

(e) Taking Breaks

If at any time while you are playing you feel the pain, take time off to do some stretches. If you watch tennis on television, you will find players who take time every now and then to stretch if they feel any pain.

Your body could only endure a certain amount of stress. Any job that requires repetitive movement has this risk of tennis elbow. Breaks allow you to minimize the possibility of tennis elbow.

(f) Icepacks

After playing sports, make sure to use an icepack on your elbows and muscles. This helps alleviate any tension that you have in your elbow and prevent the swelling that would arise. If you rest well after the game, ice and then take care of your body; you would stave off the tennis elbow effects.

(g) Warm Down After The Game

Warming down is also an important practice that should be incorporated as a habit. This gives your muscles a chance to relax and get back to its normal condition.

Once you have finished playing sports, spend some time stretching your muscles and relaxing them. Make sure that they aren't so tight. Very few people do it. You can see professional athletes doing it, but very few average people do it. Help yourself and warm down your muscles after sports.

(h) It's Not Just Sports

As mentioned in the earlier chapter, tennis elbow isn't a condition which only affects athletes. Many people who get this condition don't get it from playing sports. They merely work in jobs where repetitive arm movements are required.

Try practicing the similar techniques recommended for athletes before and after your work. Loosen up your muscles before you start work, take good breaks from work, stretch your muscles and warm down after work. Remember, you can get tennis elbow from not playing sports as well. As a matter of fact, less than forty percent of tennis elbow cases are found in athlete.

(i) See A Specialized Sports Doctor

For any time that you play a certain sport for a period of time, there is a great possibility that you would endure some sort of injury. You have a greater chance of getting the right treatment if you see a specialized sports doctor. This allows you to improve your physical condition and you get to enjoy your game.

Most common doctors just treat pain with a normal icepack and medication. However, this isn't sufficient. A doctor who is specialized in sports would follow the standard method of diagnosis. He would focus on the underlying cause rather than merely curing symptoms.

The first thing that most common doctors focus on is to relief the patient of pain, and the fastest way to do this is by medication. This is the same for surgeons. Many surgeons would just look to operate on your elbow. This is how they are being trained. Surgeons try to operate on anything that you feel a certain pain, to eliminate a problem.

The benefits of going to a doctor who specialized in sports medicine is that he is used to treating sports injuries and has different techniques of treating conditions. This ensures that the patient is able to get back to playing the sport he or she loves as quickly as possible. A good sports doctor focus on using exercises, physical therapy and other equipment to treat the patient.

Final Notes On Tennis Elbow

If you feel that you are suffering from tennis elbow, you owe it to yourself to seek out a doctor who is well trained when it comes to treating this very common condition. To ensure a swift recovery, look for a doctor who specializes in sports medicine.

From here, the doctor would prescribe a formal treatment plan that would assist you in your cure. You have to be disciplined and follow the plan thoroughly to ensure that you get the best out of the treatment. Think about the effects of not curing it and treat it as a form of motivation for you to follow through with your treatment plan.

Tennis elbow, if not treated thoroughly, would only get worst. Even if you don't feel the pain now, it would affect you in the future. Therefore, if you have a history of tennis elbow, spending time strengthening your hand is important. You not only need strength, you also need flexibility.

I hope this book has helped you understand tennis elbow better. There are things that you could do to cure and prevent it. From here, you should look for a specialized doctor. Good luck with your tennis elbow. I'm sure you can cure from tennis elbow.

Resource 1 - Tennis Elbow Secrets

Save HUNDREDS OF DOLLARS without going for physical therapy, medical equipment and consultation fees…

<u>5 Simple Steps to Eliminate Your Tennis Elbow Pain In As Little As 72 Hours and Cure It Completely Within 30 Days - Guaranteed!</u>

Find out more from:-

http://tenniselbowsecrets.wellbeingvalley.com

Resource 2 - Yoga Wellness

Stretching is an important part of curing and treating tennis elbows.

Do you want to learn basic yoga?

Want to learn how to strengthen your muscles to ensure that you wouldn't get tennis elbow?

Do You Know What Happens When You Do Yoga?

1. You can feel younger — by a decade — in only 28 days
2. You can double your energy nearly instantly
3. Your joints and connective tissue become more resilient

Want to start off with yoga fitness?

Find out more from:-

http://yogafitness.wellbeingvalley.com

CPSIA information can be obtained
at www.ICGtesting.com
Printed in the USA
BVHW032333091222
653848BV00009B/334